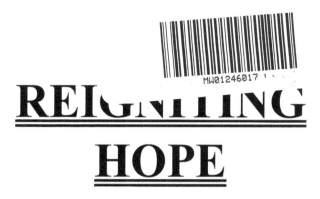

REIGNITING HOPE

HOPE

YOUR EXIT FROM DEPRESSION

Samuel Daniel

DEDICATION

This book is lovingly dedicated to my wife- the greatest woman in my life. She inspires and encourages me to be a blessing to my world.

TABLE OF CONTENTS

INTRODUCTION

Regardless of your current situation, there is hope for you. The arrows of life that hit you are the ripple effects of its envy and jealousy against your glorious future. If you have survived life's hard blows till now, I'm confident you can live on. Understand that trials, birth triumphs, tests, mother testimonies, and contests end at conquests. If you have a trial before you, picture the triumph behind it. Tests are testimonies in disguise. Moreover, the battle is hottest when the victory is near.

In 2006, the American Association of Suicidology rated suicide as the eleventh leading cause of death in America. Annually, it claimed about 33,300 lives. At the time, suicide had increased by over two hundred per cent compared to the records of the past five decades among youths between 15-24 years.

Shockingly, a report from the World Health Organization in 2021 reveals that suicide is the fourth leading cause of death among 15-29-year-olds. More disheartening is the fact that over 700,000 people commit suicide every year. We know that for every suicide, there are several suicide attempts.

You don't have to die because your time isn't up. Regardless of your circumstances, you have every reason to live your full days on earth, not in pain but hope. The fact is, every single day of your life counts. In the cumulative sense, the good times and bad you may experience are essential. There is hope for you, just as light at the end of every tunnel.

My heart goes out to those whose hearts ache. I know everyone is desperate to live, but many do not find any more reason to stay alive. In their hearts, the world has ended, the sun is set, and the dusk has overshadowed the day. This subtle lie has led countless people to the early grave. They end up causing more pain to their world than they initially felt. For everyone who committed suicide, life has not ended- they ended it abruptly. The breath in your nostrils is a constant reminder that you have hope.

Anyone who reflects on the wise words of King Solomon will continually live above the pressure to commit suicide. *"There is hope only for the living. It is better to be a live dog than a dead lion! The living at least know they will die, but the dead know nothing. They have no further reward, nor are they remembered. Whatever they did in their lifetime— loving, hating, envying—is all gone. They no longer play a part in anything here on earth. So go ahead. Eat your food with joy, and drink your wine with a happy heart, for God approves of this!"* We can only conclude on the dead. No one can tell the future of the living.

Should we be thoughtless about whatever happens to or around us? Of course, no. We all pass through different degrees of challenges. As emotional beings, we can't but express the feelings of sadness and sorrow when evil occurs. Moreover, no one is immune against the oddity of life. But our disposition to whatever happens to us matters.

Circumstances do not determine the outcome of what happens to you. The aftermath of every challenge you face is your choice. Regardless of your current predicament, scores of people have gone through similar hurdles and overcome them. If they sailed through, you can, and you will too. To assume you won't feel hurt in life is probably the greatest deception. Rest assured, you can heal from the hurt.

This book will walk you out of depression, protect your heart from hurts that stir up suicidal thoughts, and place you in the right position to rescue those considering death as an escape route. I'm happy you found this book and will help to circulate it to save ailing souls.

CHAPTER 1

UNDERSTANDING THE DEPTHS
OF DESPAIR

Despair, a formidable and overwhelming emotion, can engulf us during challenging times. It represents a profound sense of hopelessness and emptiness, leading us to believe there's no escape from our predicaments. Therefore, acknowledging the profound impact of despair is pivotal in comprehending its effects on our lives and learning to navigate its grips and depths.

First and foremost, it is crucial to recognize that despair is a regular aspect of human emotions. It is a reaction to hardship and can be brought on by trauma, loss, rejection, or failure, among other things. This complex feeling includes a combination of fear, rage, sorrow, and grief. In times of despair, hopelessness can creep in and sap one's will to make a difference.

Depression warps people's perceptions about life and tends to make them believe that there is no chance for a better future. We can negatively compare ourselves to calm people, making us feel inadequate and unworthy. This pessimistic outlook might lead to an endless circle of hopelessness.

Furthermore, it's critical to understand that despair is a variable state that varies depending on the person and the situation. While some may experience short-lived episodes, others may struggle with protracted periods that substantially negatively influence their wellbeing.

One of the toughest challenges with despair is its ability to obscure positive possibilities in our lives. It tends to overshadow the good, making breaking free from its grasp arduous. Most times, our perspective becomes skewed during difficult times. Usually, individuals require support to gain a fresh outlook at this time.

Contacting loved ones, seeing a therapist, or participating in support groups can facilitate overcoming hopelessness. These channels provide a safe environment for sharing feelings, gaining perspective, and getting advice on coping mechanisms.

Managing despair requires both seeking support and engaging in self-care. Taking care of our bodily needs, being mindful, and participating in enjoyable activities all help improve mental health. Even if these acts seem insignificant in the face of despair, they significantly affect our attitude toward life and our mood.

Importantly, it's crucial to remember that depression, like all emotions, is transient. Despite its overwhelming nature, it eventually dissipates. Cleaving to hope and reminding ourselves that things will improve can muster the strength to persevere.

Understanding the depths of despair is essential to developing coping mechanisms for this complex feeling. Even though it's a normal human sensation, it can significantly impact our lives if ignored. Seeking assistance, promoting self-care routines, and accepting hope is essential for overcoming hopelessness and building resilience. Never forget that there is always hope, even in the worst circumstances, and we are resilient enough to triumph.

Understanding Life's Undulations

"Life is like a drama. The world is the stage, people are actors, and God is the Director."

- Williams Shakespeare

One cause of damaging shock is putting absolute trust and confidence in people. When such people fail, coping with the new reality may be difficult. Life is generally like a long drama with several characters, each with a unique role.

The impacts of some people in your life will be highly beneficial but short-lived. You see some individuals walk out of your life at unexpected moments. Somehow, you must wave them goodbye and learn to survive alone as you develop new relationships.

At times, you may encounter toxic people. Unfortunately, some of them could live with you for many years. There are individuals you would be happy parting with, but somehow, they remain in your life, or something you cannot explain keeps you with them.

Everyone will always encounter good and bad individuals at different stages of their lives. This reality is inevitable. Some will make you happy, while some will make you sad. You will have loyalists and betrayers. There will be defenders and attackers in your life. As with every play, so is life: both the protagonist and the antagonist must be featured.

The diversity of life's events is what checks and balances it. Sometimes, we experience joy and, at times, sorrow. No one is immune to life's odds. We don't wish for evil, but it is sometimes inevitable. For instance, we all rejoice when a relative is delivered of a child, but we cannot stop the death of loved ones. We could pray against it, but in the long run, it is a reality we cannot avert.

I believe that our understanding and acceptance of life's swinging pendulum will help us cope with the worst it may throw against us. When someone betrays you, it is part of the drama. You learn from the experience and become more careful in investing your trust. If you run into debt or get blackmailed, you are sure to learn a lesson from it.

Anything that happens to us can teach us a lesson. Not everyone accepts this fact, but it is what it is. By remaining optimistic about life, you will maximize the potential in every experience you garner.

Suspension, not Conclusion

In drama, suspension is an essential element. Every ideal play has suspense but does not end with it. Life precisely operates the same way. There are moments of tension, worry, anxiety, uncertainty, and the like. Looking back, you will admit you have overcome many of these seasons. There were times of hopelessness that you sailed through. You have escaped several death traps you can't help but be grateful for.

Whatever difficult season you are going through is suspense, not the end of your life. Life itself is not meant to end in suspense. Sadly, many assume suspension as the conclusion and end their lives abruptly. Meanwhile, today's mess can form the message for tomorrow. If you endure the challenges of today, you will enjoy the chances of tomorrow.

A king accidentally lost the hallux on his right leg while hunting with one of his servants. The servant attempted to console him to no avail. He complained bitterly and lashed God for being so dumb in rescuing him. The servant upheld that there is a purpose for whatever happens and that the king should be grateful for life. Instead of being soothed, the king got infuriated and incarcerated the servant.

After healing up, the king went for another hunting game alone. This time, some ritualists abducted him. After conjuring some diabolic forces, he was unfit for the sacrifice because of the amputation of his toe. The abductors released him, and he returned home rejoicing for his deliverance. Then, he remembered the words of his servant.

The king believes that whatever happens to anyone has a purpose, but he could not reconcile why he had to punish the servant for an offense he never committed. When the king got to his palace, he called for the servant and shared his ordeals with him. He appreciated God for allowing him to lose his hallux before the abduction.

But the king turned to the servant and asked: "If everything has a purpose, why did I imprison you unjustly?" The servant smiled and said: "I would be the perfect sacrifice for the ritual had I gone hunting with you."

We must consider our life experiences cumulatively before we can judge accurately. You cannot conclude your life based on a bitter experience. People who do so need to be more confident and able to see what the future holds for them. You don't judge a whole play by a scene. Do you?

Never take suspense as the end of your life. Your life is like a drama. The world is the stage, with many actors, but God is the Director. You cannot assume the Director's position as an actor. The script of your life has not been concluded, so don't assume.

Many people are like the king in our story. They soon give up on life. They insult God and shut good people out of their lives when the slightest challenge comes. Soon, they are left alone, and the feeling of loneliness begins to creep into their souls. This is how many have altered the scripts they ought to have acted in life. They have taken the Director's position and got everything messed up in no time.

Follow the Pace

Your life is not yours, so you can't control it. We will hardly avoid ruin until we allow the Creator to reform our lives. You must have observed that certain situations are beyond human control. This means there is a Director of all things—God.

Well, you may wish to blame humanity's predicament on God because He is the Director of life, but that would be stark ignorance. Human errors induce certain events, and some happen naturally. Whatever the case, God has a way of turning your tests into testimonies and trials into triumphs. But this happens only when He takes the lead, and you follow the pace.

You may have a little beginning and a rough process, but your end will be great. Your life experience might have been terrible, but don't conclude yet. Every drama features different scenes. In the same way, you will experience different seasons in your life.

All through the year, we experience seasonal variations in weather conditions. But we have learnt the coping strategies for the winter, summer, autumn and spring. Although we feel differently each season, we are optimistic there will be changes. Some seasons are difficult to cope with- the extreme heat or cold, for instance. But seasons change with time. Life is calibrated into seasons. You will watch your bad times fade as you wait patiently and stay positive.

In the academic world, there is a calendar that governs the length of time you are to spend in each class. Before you graduate to a new level, you are mandated to write promotional exams. Some tests, trials, and challenges we face are life's promotional examinations. They are real practical issues, but we get stronger and better as we endure and learn from them.

History has shown that people overcoming more challenges have greater social relevance. If they had given up or committed suicide, they would have died unnoticed as mere men. But their resilience gave them a voice after they've departed from the world. Those who stay alive are not people without challenges, and those who call it quits and resort to suicide are not the most embattled people.

In the words of Robert Schuller, "tough times never last, but tough people do." Moreover, only the tough gets going when the going gets tough. We have the weakness to call it quits in the race of life but the strength to pull through when it seems life is not worth living.

Your living is beyond you. Whether you believe it or not, you are someone's source of inspiration. You are not alive for yourself alone. Other destinies connect to yours. So, you contribute more to your world than you've ever thought, heard, or known. Someone needs you to survive. If you commit murder, many things will die.

CHAPTER 2

HOW DEPRESSION LIES TO YOU

Depression is not only a mental illness; rather, it is an overwhelming shadow that warps our sense of reality and functions more like a cunning manipulator. This chapter explores the many ways that depression lies to us, and how important it is to identify these lies as we set out on the path to recovery.

Fundamentally, depression feeds on lies. It takes advantage of our weaknesses, thrives on illogical ideas, and convinces us that it is the only version of reality that is both limited and gloomy. This kind of deception frequently leads to an unbreakable downward spiral in one's thinking. But the first step in recovering our truths and, eventually, our lives, is admitting these lies.

Common Lies Told by Depression

1. "You're Alone"

One of the most insidious lies depression tells is that you're isolated in your suffering. It isolates you from friends, family, and even yourself. This solitude often triggers the belief that no one can understand your pain, which spurs feelings of hopelessness. In reality, countless people have experienced similar struggles, and many are willing to lend a listening ear or a comforting presence.

2. "You're Defective"

Depression frequently persuades you that your difficulties are evidence of your own shortcomings or failures. You can think that you are a burden to other people and feel damaged, imperfect, or undeserving. This myth obscures the reality that mental health issues are widespread and do not determine your value as a person, encouraging feelings of guilt and despair.

3. "Nothing Will Change"

Permanence mythology is yet another potent fabrication. When you're depressed, it might seem like nothing will get better, which makes you give up and do nothing. But not only is change feasible, it's frequently a necessary step in the healing process. A person's viewpoint and attitude can significantly improve with the help of supportive networks, lifestyle modifications, and techniques.

4. "Everything Is Your Fault"

Depression frequently makes you believe that you are to blame for all of your issues. It distorts reality by emphasizing errors and ignoring successes. This internalized blame makes it harder to view circumstances objectively by intensifying feelings of shame and self-loathing. Self-compassion is essential, and we must acknowledge that errors are a part of life and do not determine who we are or how valuable we are.

5. "You Don't Deserve Help"

Many people who struggle with depression harbor the underlying idea that they are undeserving of love, attention, or support. This kind of thinking might keep you from asking for assistance, which feeds the loneliness and hopelessness cycle. Recall that asking for assistance is a brave step toward recovery and self-empowerment rather than a sign of weakness.

The first step is to recognize the frequent lies that sadness tells us. The true difficulty is figuring out when such lies start to enter our minds. Maintaining a diary, consulting with reliable friends, or getting expert assistance can help to establish a framework that is supportive in recognizing harmful distortions and swapping them out for kind and accurate affirmations.

Reframing Your Thought Patterns

It's critical to deliberately reframe such beliefs as soon as you recognize the lies that depression tells you. Techniques from cognitive behavioral therapy (CBT) may be helpful in this process. You may start to loosen depression's hold on your mind by confronting negative ideas and rephrasing them into more achievable, affirmative claims. For example, you may phrase it like this: "I have people who care about me, even if I don't always feel it," as opposed to thinking, "I'm all alone." This change in viewpoint begins to create a bridge that leads back to connection and optimism.

Building Your Toolkit

It's invaluable to arm yourself with tools to combat these lies as they arise. These tools may include:

- **Mindfulness Techniques**: Practicing mindfulness can help ground you in the present moment, making it easier to observe your thoughts without judgment.

- **Cognitive Behavioral Exercises**: Engage in exercises designed to challenge and reframe negative ideas and thoughts.

- **Support Networks**: Surround yourself with well-meaning friends, family, or support groups who can remind you of the truths you may struggle to see.

- **Professional Guidance**: Don't hesitate to reach out to mental health professionals. They can provide you with strategies tailored to your individual needs and guide you on your healing journey.

Although depression's falsehoods are crafty, they don't have complete control over you. It is essential to identify these lies and take proactive measures to refute them if you want to build resilience and get well. You possess the resilience to look past the mask that depression puts on your life and move back toward connection, hope, and recovery.

CHAPTER 3

EMBRACING POSITIVITY IN THE FACE OF DESPONDENCY

"The real reason for not committing suicide is because you always know how swell life gets again after the hell is over."

— Ernest Hemingway

Yes! Change is the only constant. Nature consistently reminds us that nothing is permanent but change. Seasons change. The weather fluctuates mysteriously; even some living organisms' life cycles are fascinating. Consider a butterfly, for instance. What you admire as a beautifully feathered butterfly was once a creeping caterpillar. It inches and crawls around by squeezing its muscles and undulating in sequences.

Though helpless and frail, the caterpillar needs time to begin to fly. As it continues to feed, in a few weeks, the caterpillar metamorphoses into a new form and begins to fly. What a change! This is precisely what happens in our lives.

You didn't start to walk and run the following month after your birth. The toddling days were a necessary part of your growth. Those physical processes could sometimes be invisible in other areas of our lives. There are times when you may have to crawl through life. Such an experience may be associated with pain, but you must see it as a process. The caterpillar does not need to be frustrated because it only passes through a process. It needed to crawl before flying.

You will stay positive if you see every challenge before you as a process leading you to a greater height. Those who looked down on you when you were crawling will soon look up to you when you begin to fly. Your pain is part of the process leading to your glorious destination. You have to endure it and be unapologetic about it. You will fly after you have crept.

The Furnace of Fire

"But he knows where I am going. And when he tests me, I will come out as pure as gold."

- Job

No one appreciates gold in its crude form; it requires fire for its transformation. Fire unveils its beauty and value. The more it is heated, the more it glitters. You are probably in the furnace of life because you are determined to be gold.

Trials do to us what fire does to gold. Job concluded that when life's challenges test him, he will come out of the furnace as pure as gold. This is the greatest motivation for life. Furnaces are not playing grounds, but you can stay positive while being refined. You will never come out of a challenge worse than you got into it, except if you give up.

For Job, there were not multiple ideas; the only thought flowing through his mind was that he would come out of his predicament refined. You won't ever get defeated with such a mindset. Accepting defeat is succumbing to a negative mindset. If you stay positive, your challenges will force out the best in you.

Job is a typical example of one that should have an excuse for committing suicide. Yet, he was hopeful, optimistic, and motivated. Today, his experience strengthens us to keep our hopes alive despite the storms raging against us.

The First Trial

Job's unpleasant experience began after a conversation that was held behind him. Amazingly, God dialogued with Satan over Job's life. He initiated the discussion by asking whether the devil had seen and observed Job's righteousness and uprightness. As you know, the devil is an unrepentant enemy. He tried to argue with God by explaining why Job seemed to love Him.

The conversation got heated, and God and Satan signed a deal. Before then, there was an invisible wall of protection around Job and his family. He was the wealthiest man in the East. He was god-fearing, rich, and famous. But, to prove a point, the devil asked God to allow him to deal with Job. "Deal! Do whatever pleases you with what he has, but don't touch him," God affirmed.

You can trust the devil when it comes to damaging things. He has no other occupation than stealing, killing, and destroying. Satan left God's presence with a warrant to destroy and make things go bizarre for Job's family.

Shortly after that, unimaginable catastrophes began to befall Job.

On a fateful day, Job lost all that he had. First, one of his servants reported that the Sabeans attacked them on the farm while ploughing with the oxen. The invaders took away all the oxen and the asses that were feeding beside them. Only the servant who brought the report to Job escaped; others died.

As the first servant broke the bad news to Job, one of his shepherds hopped in. He reported that a mysterious fire came down from heaven and consumed all the sheep with every other servant. Only he was the survivor.

While the second servant was relating his ordeal, the third servant rushed in. He told Job that some Chaldeans had attacked them and stolen all the camels they were tending. Other servants were killed, but he escaped.

The first three evil reports were not as disheartening as the last one. While the third servant spoke, the fourth came in with the saddest news. He explained how a strong wind from the wilderness blew against the house where Job's children were feasting, and it collapsed, killing them all. Job had ten children— seven sons and three daughters. He lost all his livestock and children in a day. What situation can be worse than this?

Like any other human, Job responded to the evil scenarios by rending his clothes and shaving his head. Those were conspicuous signs of mourning in ancient times. However, Job worshipped God immediately. He admitted that God gives and takes away. He never said anything against God. Was he pained? Absolutely! We know this by his physical reaction when he tore his clothes and shaved his head. They were signs he was humiliated.

We can't be thoughtless about the things that happen to us. But we can control our reactions. Job was not less or more of a human than any of us is. I wonder how many thoughts would be flowing through his heart then. Everything he had was gone, but he never despaired.

The Second Trial

I hope you remember that Job's ordeal was the result of a deal between God and Satan. At the end of the first trial, Satan was disappointed to see Job standing firm, remaining loyal to God, and being optimistic about life. Listen, the devil laughs when you cry and wear a long face. But he feels disappointed when he throws challenges at you, and you smile through them.

Satan aimed to make Job depressed and despaired until he renounced God. But he met his waterloo when Job bowed in worship to God. You must be determined to whip the devil whenever he comes around you. He is tireless and will always raise his ugly head. So, you must position yourself right against his assaults.

Another day came when God boasted about Job's integrity to Satan. This time, he brought up a stronger argument. "Skin for skin! A man will give up everything to save his life. But reach out and take away his health, and he will surely curse you to your face," Satan argued. "Do whatever pleases you to him, but you have no authority over his life," God responded.

You see, Satan has no authority to take your life. He can afflict you at worst, but your life is in God's hands. I believe that God does not give you the authority to take your life, too. If God restricted Satan from taking Job's life, then you cannot decide to commit suicide. The breath in your nostrils is not yours or Satan's. Neither of you have authority over it but God. Satan wants to bring calamity into people's lives and afflict them.

Finally, Satan struck Job with a terrible boil from head to foot. It was a pathetic condition for Job, who declined from the limelight into obscurity. It seemed that Job's sun began to set while it was still day. To alleviate the pains of his boil, he sat among the ashes and scrapped his skin with a piece of broken pottery.

Human Reactions

Your experiences are indeed exclusive to you. People cannot fully comprehend the weight of pain you bear over some issues. Unfortunately, their judgment of you can be sincerely wrong. Even if someone has had your experience, their pain sensitivity cannot be the same as yours.

For instance, two women may lose their husbands at different intervals. Although what they lost is the same, the effect on the two of them can never be exact. The first woman might have raised her children to a reasonable life height and lived with her husband for over thirty years. But the second woman might have lived less than a decade with her husband and had a lot of responsibility to raise her young kids. In this case, you expect them to feel different levels of pain for losing the same thing.

In the same scenario, some circumstances could make the older woman feel more pain than the younger one. The younger woman, for instance, might have suffered in an abusive marriage for about a decade. If her husband dies, she may step into a season of healing and refreshing. But for the older woman with a long-term intimate relationship with her husband, saying goodbye could be the hardest thing for her.

These analogies help us understand that we do not know exactly how people feel when they experience difficult times. So, we cannot judge them for acting in certain ways. Even if you had a similar experience with someone, you can only have an idea of what they are going through within them. Therefore, our words and reactions should bring healing to their ailing hearts.

When Satan saw that Job did not lose his integrity with God, he stirred up his wife to counsel him to curse God and die. For Job's wife, death was better than pain and humiliation. Observably, what you say to a depressed individual has weight. It can either energize or enervate the person in question. Several people's conditions have worsened because of unhealthy words from folks around them.

But, you see, Job was an exceptional man. He never heeded his wife's counsel to curse God. He did not despair. He knew that a living dog was better than a dead lion.

Job's three friends came to console him, and for seven days, they were dumbfounded. None of them could speak a word when they saw his physical state. "What else could be responsible for such a demotion from grace to grass?" they wondered. Finally, everyone concluded that Job was a sinner with whom nemesis had caught up. They accused him of wickedness and chastised him with words.

Hope helps you cope

In 1873, Horatio G. Spafford and his family scheduled travel to Europe from the United States. He was held back due to some pressing business. However, his wife and daughters boarded the French liner *Ville du Havre* and travelled ahead of him. On November 22, the ship collided with the English ship *Lochearn* and sank in twelve minutes.

Unfortunately, this tragic event claimed several lives, including Mr. Spafford's four daughters. Finally arriving in Wales, Mrs Spafford, the only survivor in the Spaffords' family, cabled her husband: "Saved alone." Hearing the news, Spafford boarded a boat to meet his wife, and close to the scene of the tragic event on the high sea, he wrote the famous hymn: *"When peace like a river attendeth my way, when sorrows like sea billows roll; whatever my lot, thou hast taught me to say, "It is well, it is well with my soul."*

D. L. Moody, a close friend, visited the Spaffords in England upon hearing the news and reported him saying, "It is well; the will of God be done." Later, Philip Bliss, another friend of the Spaffords, wrote the tune of the hymnal text written by Spafford, which was finally published in 1876.

In 1871, before Spafford wrote his famous text, he had recorded a heavy loss in the Chicago fire outbreak. This event was followed by the death of his four daughters two years later. Sadly, the family lost their son in 1880. Like Job's friends, some unkind church members where Spafford served as a Sunday school teacher and a trustee for the Presbyterian Theological Seminary accused him of suffering for his secret sins.

Spafford and his wife left Chicago for Jerusalem in 1881 with some friends, and he founded an American colony there. In later years, Bertha Spafford Vester, another daughter of the Spaffords, told their family story, which she tagged: *"Our Jerusalem."*

Today, many are spurred to sing Mr. Spafford's hymn when they are happy. However, it was the outpouring of a man's soul in the most traumatizing years of his life. It is interesting to hear of people who passed through difficult situations and finally left their impacts on the sand of time. People are attracted to the glory, not to the story. I believe that we are not more of saints than Spafford or Job, neither were they more of sinners than we.

Job's story is not fictitious; several religions believe and teach it. Although some may doubt the sequence of Job's predicament and argue that such a coincidence could not perfectly align with real life, Spafford's story is similar to Job's. These stories are not folktales. If these men could survive their dark and tragic seasons, you have greater hope than they.

Job could cope with his challenging times because he never lost hope. It is difficult to find anyone whose situation is worse than Job's. He lost not only his material possessions but all his children. His wife preferred to give him over to death, and his friends were antagonistic. There was almost nothing left for him than hope.

No matter what you are going through today, several people have had worse experiences and overcome them. Think about the Spaffords. How were they able to keep their heads above the waters? The answer is not far-fetched: they trusted and hoped in God. This hope does not make anyone ashamed. It brings refreshing to your soul. You have every reason to live and be full of hope.

Behind the Scene

Nothing happens accidentally. The law of cause and effect governs life. Our ignorance of the cause of events cannot disprove it. An invisible force engineers every physical circumstance. This understanding will illuminate your heart.

Let's get back to Job. He was probably having a pleasant time with his family when God began to call Satan's attention to him. He was utterly ignorant of what was happening behind his life's scenes. But decisions were made about him, and they played out exactly as planned.

In a nutshell, Job suffered all to prove a point- his loyalty. God allowed Satan to afflict him, not because He was inconsiderate, but for His great confidence in Job. Satan, on the other side, thought he knew how exactly to make Job suffer till he renounced God. Job's ordeal began when God cast his vote of confidence on him.

Job did not suffer for committing any atrocity. He was only being tried. Amazingly, God didn't prepare his heart for such a trial. Even if Job had sinned, I believe other sinners in his days never had his experiences. You could be going through trials, too. An argument might have ensued behind you, and the effect is the only thing you see. If that is the case, hold on. You will come out triumphantly.

What you do in the season of trials is noteworthy. Job overcame, and today, we can tell his story. When you overcome, others will read your story and find strength and hope for their lives. If Job had committed suicide, the devil would have won on that account. You can decide not to let the devil take the praise or win the victory over your life.

The end will speak

No matter what life throws at you, if you are optimistic, you will end positively. In the process of time, everyone becomes what they believe. People who pitch their tents in the negative side of life will never find comfort and joy. Their pessimism is a choice they made, and life would honor it. But when your belief system is positive, regardless of your pains in life, your end will reflect what you truly believe.

With all that bedeviled Job, glaringly, he remained hopeful. "If people die, can they come back to life? But I will wait for better times, wait till this time of trouble is ended," he said. Job knew that waiting brings healing. He was sure that the season of trouble would expire. With hope, he waited to see the end and saw it gloriously. Job did not die miserably. He recovered all his losses in double-folds.

Job 42:12-13 summarizes the end of Job's life thus: "The Lord blessed the last part of Job's life even more than he had blessed the first. Job owned 14,000 sheep, 6,000 camels, 2,000 head of cattle, and 1000 donkeys. He was the father of seven sons and three daughters" (NLT).

No one can predict the future of the living; only the dead is hopeless. A tree cut down has hope. If its roots remain in the ground, it will sprout and bud again. If you have suffered loss, it's time to embrace recovery. Regardless of what you have lost, you can find healing and restoration.

Embrace Positivity

Life's journey often presents unforeseen challenges, creating constant obstacles that leave us feeling overwhelmed and disheartened. Amidst this turmoil, negativity easily seeps in, especially when circumstances appear unfavorable.

Nevertheless, amidst despair, it's vital to recognize our capability to choose our outlook. We hold the power to dwell on adversities or adopt a positive perspective, finding ways to surmount these challenges. Though embracing positivity amid despondency may prove demanding, it remains achievable and transformative in our lives.

The primary step toward embracing positivity involves acknowledging and embracing our emotions. It's natural to experience despondency periodically, and permitting ourselves to feel these emotions is crucial. Instead of suppressing or disregarding negativity, fully embracing these feelings allows us to comprehend and progress through them.

Once we've acknowledged our emotions, redirecting our focus toward positivity becomes essential. This may involve actively pursuing optimistic thoughts and experiences. Cultivating gratitude through practices like daily reflections on three things to be thankful for or appreciating the beauty in our surroundings initiates this shift.

Additionally, surrounding ourselves with positive influences plays a pivotal role. The company we keep significantly shapes our mindset. Encircling ourselves with encouraging and hopeful individuals offers a fresh outlook, empowering us to confront and transcend challenges.

Recognizing challenges and setbacks as integral parts of life, opportunities for personal growth rather than impediments signifies a profound shift in perspective. Embracing these instances as avenues for learning cultivates resilience and alters how we approach difficulties.

Moreover, physical and mental self-care facilitates the embrace of positivity. Engaging in activities that bring joy, practising mindfulness, or incorporating exercise into our routine elevates mood and overall wellbeing.

A sense of purpose and direction in life also contributes significantly to embracing positivity. Goals, no matter how small or large, provide motivation and foster a positive mindset, propelling us forward.

Adopting a positive mindset might seem insurmountable in the face of despondency. However, we can gradually shift our attitude toward a more positive outlook by acknowledging emotions, actively seeking positivity, surrounding ourselves with support, altering perspectives on challenges, practising self-care, and nurturing a sense of purpose.

It's not about dismissing issues or pretending perfection but harnessing strength and resilience to grow and triumph over them. Embracing positivity amidst despondency demands effort, but its rewards are immeasurable.

CHAPTER 4

SHIFTING YOUR MINDSET

A person's deeply entrenched attitudes and ideas about themselves and their skills are referred to as their mindset. Our views and responses to our experiences are shaped by these ideas. A pessimistic outlook can send those suffering from depression into an unending circle of hopelessness, despair, and self-doubt. The first step in ending this loop is to intentionally change our perspective.

Our mentality is one of the most effective weapons we have while trying to overcome depression. Our perception and interaction with our thoughts, feelings, and the environment have a profound effect on our emotional health. This chapter will look at doable tactics to change your perspective and give your life back to you.

The Impact of Negative Self-Talk

One of the most prevalent obstacles to mental wellness is negative self-talk. Phrases like "I'm a burden to others," "I'll never feel better," and "I'm not good enough" contribute to emotions of worthlessness and loneliness. Identifying these mental patterns is the first step towards making a change. By challenging and substituting positive affirmations for these negative narratives, journaling your thoughts may be a useful tool for bringing attention to these ideas.

Practicing Self-Compassion

The greatest significant change we can make is to become more self-compassionate. It entails being nice and understanding to ourselves as we would be toward a friend. We may accept our sentiments and acknowledge our problems instead of judging ourselves for having depression. A kinder inner dialogue can be fostered by methods like self-compassion meditation or guided imagery, which can help to mend the wounds caused by a poor self-perception.

Reframing Negative Thoughts

A cognitive-behavioral strategy called reframing entails altering our perspective on events and circumstances. We may use setbacks as chances for learning and progress rather than seeing them as failures. When confronted with difficult ideas, consider these questions:

- What evidence do I have for or against this thought?

- Is this thought really true, or is it an exaggeration?

- How would I advise a friend in a similar situation?

By cultivating this level of introspection, you can start to replace detrimental thoughts with more constructive ones.

Gratitude and Positivity

Gratitude is an attitude that may be transformed through cultivation. Research has indicated that emphasizing the good parts of our lives might improve our mood and lessen depressive symptoms. Begin by recording three things each day for which you are grateful in a gratitude diary. You may change your attention from what is wrong in your life to what is good by adopting this easy exercise.

Embracing Mindfulness

Another effective strategy for changing your perspective is mindfulness, which is the practice of being present in the moment without passing judgment. By engaging in mindfulness practices, we may better monitor our thoughts and feelings without being overwhelmed. Deep breathing exercises and guided meditations are two examples of mindfulness practices that can help you become more grounded and less ruminative, which is a typical symptom of depression.

Building a Growth Mindset

The idea that intelligence and ability can be increased through hard work and persistence is known as a growth mindset. By cultivating a development mentality, we can face difficulties head-on rather than giving up. Establish modest, doable objectives and acknowledge your progress. This strategy not only boosts motivation but also strengthens the conviction that change is achievable.

Seeking Support

When you're not alone, it's usually easier to change your perspective. Making connections with others, whether they be friends, family, or support networks, may offer the accountability and encouragement that is required in trying times. Emotional burdens can be lessened and a feeling of community can be fostered via sharing ideas and personal experiences.

One of the most important steps on the path to depression rehabilitation is changing your perspective. The benefits of increased emotional health and resilience outweigh the time and effort required. You may change your inner story, inspire hope, and rekindle your enthusiasm for life by using the techniques and skills covered in this chapter. Recall that every action you do, no matter how tiny, puts you one step closer to a better future. Accept the process and allow yourself to develop.

CHAPTER 5

STRATEGIES FOR CONQUERING DEPRESSION

Globally, depression is a prevalent mental health issue that impacts a substantial population. It seems to be a profound, persistent pessimism, depression, and lack of interest in once-enjoyable activities.

People become despondent when it seeps into their spirits and undermines their self-worth over time. In actuality, depression lowers people's quality of life and exerts a negative mental impact on them. People who dwell in despair and melancholy ultimately mirror the negative ideas and circumstances that they encounter. On the other hand, optimism is a lubricant that lessens the frictional consequences of life.

Despite the crippling effects of depression, there are useful strategies that might help people overcome it and find fulfillment again. These useful tactics will aid in the fight against depression and the symptoms that go along with it.

Seek for Help

"To anyone out there who's hurting — it's not a sign of weakness to ask for help. It's a sign of strength."

- Barack Obama

Deeply, the stigma associated with mental illness keeps individuals from asking for assistance. Occasionally, it could transform into the anxiety of being perceived negatively or misinterpreted. Whatever the cause, it's time to end the stigma and acknowledge how critical it is to get treatment when depressed.

The quickest path to depression is to repress emotional distress. Basically, people need to realize that sadness is neither a moral failing nor a show of weakness. Like any other ailment, it's a medical problem that has to be properly treated. Enough said, depression is treatable.

Depression may be brought on by a number of things, either separately or in combination. A mix of biological, psychological, environmental, and hereditary variables may be involved. It is difficult to ignore or treat depression with optimistic thinking alone. For this reason, getting expert assistance is essential to controlling and recovering from depression.

having help has several benefits, one of which is having a proper diagnosis and course of therapy for depression. Depression symptoms can vary greatly from person to person and take many distinct forms. Merely a mental health professional is qualified to identify depression and provide a personalized treatment strategy.

This might entail treatment, medication, support groups, and lifestyle changes, depending on how serious the issue is. If depression is not addressed, it can worsen and lead to more issues with both mental and physical health.

Additionally, getting treatment for depression might make you feel validated and relieved. Many individuals who suffer from depression believe that no one else can relate to their situation, which makes them feel alone and lonely. But if you ask for assistance, you'll find that you're not alone.

Mental health professionals are adept at listening to patients without passing judgment and providing a safe, supportive space for them to express their thoughts and feelings. This encouragement and affirmation may go a long way toward helping someone who is depressed feel heard and understood.

Another important reason to get therapy for depression is to keep it from interfering with your day-to-day activities. When you're sad, it can be hard to focus, do everyday tasks, and maintain relationships. This might lead to problems in relationships, the workplace, and education. Early intervention, however, can help you acquire coping skills to manage your symptoms and help you prevent the negative impacts of depression. Once more, getting treatment for depression is a courageous and commendable step. It takes courage and bravery to admit when you need assistance and to take the required actions to enhance your mental health. You are taking control of your life and making positive changes when you ask for assistance. It is a sign of self-care and self-love, which are essential to enhancing mental health.

When you're depressed, it's important to get treatment for your physical and emotional well-being. It is a step toward healing and rehabilitation, not a show of weakness. Never consider yourself to be alone yourself. Many people care about you and can support your healing. So don't be embarrassed to seek for assistance.

If you think you or someone you know is depressed, get guidance and support from a mental health professional. Asking for assistance is the first step in leading a happy and full life. You're worthy of that.

Embrace Self-Care

In today's hectic and stressful world, many people frequently experience overload and burnout. Given the constant pressure to balance their duties to their families, jobs, and personal lives, it should not be surprising that a significant portion of the population suffers from mental health issues like depression.

While there are numerous possibilities for treatment, self-care is a strategy that is often overlooked. Embracing self-care is a powerful anti-depressant tactic.

Self-care goes beyond treating oneself to special meals or pleasures once in a while. It takes intentional work to put your mental, emotional, and physical health first. It entails looking after your physical, emotional, and spiritual needs in all facets of your life. It involves realizing your wants and acting to satisfy them.

So why is self-care so important in the battle against depression? It's not absurd to conclude that grief weakens a person's sense of value and self-worth. It can make someone feel exhausted, overwhelmed, and powerless. Nonetheless, self-care may support the development of a sense of worth and compassion for oneself as well as assist fight these negative emotions.

When we make time for self-care, it helps reduce stress and anxiety, which enables us to better handle the challenges and obligations of daily life. Spending time outside or practicing mindfulness meditation can assist promote mental serenity and reduce stress and anxiety. Additionally, engaging in pleasurable and fulfilling hobbies or interests might help ward off melancholy thoughts and sensations.

Given the close relationship between mental and physical health, self-care is just as important in fostering physical wellness. A balanced diet, consistent exercise, and adequate sleep are all crucial components of self-care that can improve overall wellbeing. It has been shown that exercise is an effective way to reduce depression symptoms. Endorphins are feel-good chemicals released as a result of it, which can improve mood and diminish depressed and hopeless sentiments.

Additionally, self-care can improve social networks and interpersonal interactions, which is advantageous for depressed people. Taking care of oneself may contribute to our emotional well-being and increase our capacity to resolve conflicts and issues in our relationships. It also helps us to establish appropriate boundaries and prioritize our needs, which may lead to more fulfilling and supportive relationships.

Individuals who take care of themselves can recover their sense of autonomy and mastery over their life. Even while depression often leaves sufferers feeling overwhelmed and powerless, self-care techniques can help them restore a sense of control. When we put our welfare first—which we can accomplish by taking care of ourselves—we can feel more in control of our lives.

Most importantly, remember that taking care of oneself is not selfish; rather, it is a necessary component of self-preservation. As a result, don't undervalue the significance of self-care if you're depressed. Make time for your wellbeing and witness the benefits it may bring to your mental health. Never forget that you cannot pour from an empty cup, so take care of yourself first.

Knowing when and how to avoid individuals and situations that heighten melancholy, despair, and poor self-esteem is a part of practicing self-care. Trying to impress people comes with a risk of self-harm. Self-care maintains your heart full of love and hope and protects you from emotional jabs.

Eat a healthy diet, get enough sleep to prevent burnout, and regularly partake in enjoyable physical activity and other activities that encourage contentment and relaxation. Take time to pamper yourself and learn how to treat yourself. These customs successfully raise wellness and elevate mood.

Challenge Negative Thought Patterns

Nobody ever becomes depressed unless their way of thinking is changed. While there are many causes of depression, all victims experience a similar symptom of negativity occasionally. People ponder suicide when these feelings get worse because they no longer feel hopeful.

Anyone recovering from depressed trauma may experience a period of transitory negative thinking. The essence of life might be destroyed if improperly managed. At this point, I've discovered that a lot of people just focus on and perceive the bad aspects of life.

I remember counselling a lady who thought her relationship wouldn't work out. She accumulated a lot of falsehoods in her mind, and they dictated her reaction to life and her fiancé. Her past failed relationships were affecting her current friendship. The past remained present with her, and she thought, felt, reasoned, and behaved like her past.

The lady in question never complained about her new fiancé. She had always been the problem. She nurtured the thought the guy would someday leave her like others, and the thought ate deep into her until she got frustrated and considered committing suicide.

Many people cook and serve themselves lies when they allow negative thoughts to perch on their minds. They assume things that are not real and believe in them so much that they form a stronghold in their hearts.

Our thinking greatly influences our emotions and actions. Negative thoughts can set off a chain reaction of unfavorable feelings and actions that might eventually contribute to the onset of depression. For this reason, breaking destructive thought patterns is essential to treating depression.

However, how do unfavorable mental habits start? They may result from genetics, traumas, social pressures, or past experiences. Identifying and addressing the harmful thought patterns we've formed is critical, regardless of the underlying cause. The first step in altering them is this.

The good news is that negative thought patterns can be changed. It takes time and effort, but it is a powerful strategy in combating depression. Here are some practical ways to reverse negative thought patterns and take control of your life:

#*Practice self-awareness*

But how can negative thought patterns begin? Genetics, traumatic experiences, social forces, or even prior experiences could be the cause. We must recognize and deal with the negative thought patterns we have developed, regardless of the root cause. This is the first step towards changing them.

For instance, you recount your thoughts, actions, and reactions at the close of each day before you sleep. This will help you to evaluate how much of your actions and reactions were prompted by evil thoughts. If you notice a particular style of negativity, note it and develop strategies to deal with it.

#*Challenge your thoughts*

Challenge your negative thoughts as soon as you become aware of them. Consider whether these are presumptions or based on actual information. Our unfavorable perceptions of a situation are often more grounded in our minds than in fact. We can recast our ideas more optimistically and groundedly by confronting them.

In the case of the lady I counselled, her perception ruled over actual reality. She almost ruined her marital relationship until she learned how to challenge her thoughts and grow beyond her past.

#*Practice positive self-talk*

Our internal discourse greatly impacts our mental health. Rather than always criticizing ourselves, we ought to engage in constructive self-talk. This entails deliberately swapping out negative ideas for optimistic ones. For instance, state, "I am capable and resilient" rather than "I'm a failure."

Every action emanates from the thought realm. If you can be positively conscious, you can take charge of your life. Every positive word you speak to yourself breaks down the walls of negativity in your life. Eventually, your confession becomes your possession and reality.

#*Surround yourself with positivity*

Confessions of gratitude are insufficient. The kind of individuals we spend time with can also impact the way we think. Embrace a positive and encouraging circle of people who will lift you up and help you see the good in everything. Spend as little time as possible with people who depress you or make you think negatively.

Avoid people who magnify your weaknesses and shortcomings. As you practice positive self-talk, complement your effort with positive people. As you speak positivity from within and you hear the same from without, your life reechoes optimism and reverberates joy.

#Seek professional help

Changing negative thought patterns can be challenging, and it is okay to seek help. A therapist or counsellor can provide the necessary tools and support to challenge and change your negative thought patterns effectively.

Freeing oneself from negative thoughts takes time, patience, and consistent effort. But the benefits are well worth it. By changing our negative thought patterns, we can reduce the intensity and frequency of depressive episodes. We can also improve our mental well-being and lead more fulfilling lives.

When we become aware of negative thoughts, we can end the vicious cycle of negativity and fight depression by actively challenging them and replacing them with positive ones. Never forget that you are in charge of your mental well-being and can alter the way you think. Thus, begin today and change your perspective to one that is healthier and more optimistic.

Cultivate a Support Network

A support network is a collection of people who offer emotional, mental, physical, and even spiritual support during trying times. These people could be members of your social group, family, friends, or coworkers. Having a support system is essential, mainly when depression is present.

Feeling alone and isolated is one of the most unpleasant realities of depression. A support system can assist in fighting negative emotions by offering emotional support. Those in your support system are there to listen, console, and lend a shoulder when needed. They can also assist you in adopting a fresh viewpoint and guide you in overcoming the difficulties associated with depression.

Depression can make you feel alienated even in the company of friends and family. On the other hand, a support system might help you feel accepted and at home. Knowing that there are people who love and support you can help you feel less alone and more confident. You feel more secure in a group of kind friends and family members.

A network of supporters offers accountability and spurs one to persevere. A friend in your support system could go with you to appointments or assist you in maintaining a self-care schedule, for instance. You may need that extra motivation to keep moving forward when you realize someone depends on you.

Furthermore, it is not unusual for depressed individuals to resort to unhealthy coping mechanisms like substance misuse or social distancing. A support system, however, can motivate you to take up healthy coping strategies, including working out, going to therapy, or spending time with close friends and family. To prevent relapse, they can also assist you in identifying triggers and offer support.

A strong social network can offer more than just emotional support—it can also be helpful in several other ways. This might be preparing meals, running errands, or helping with child care. Having assistance with regular duties can be quite beneficial when suffering from depression, as it can feel overwhelming at times.

For several people, talking to close ones about depression might be difficult since they might not comprehend what you're going through. Conversely, a social network's supportive role fosters a secure environment where you can express your emotions without worrying about being judged. This can help you process your feelings and be quite therapeutic.

Developing a robust support system proves immensely beneficial in overcoming depression. Whether through family, friends, or support groups, surrounding oneself with understanding and supportive individuals is essential. Openly discussing feelings with trusted confidants lessens feelings of isolation and provides comfort and validation.

Remember, you are not meant to go through dark times alone. We are social beings; we can't live independently of ourselves. Someone needs you to survive, and you need others to lean on, too. Don't bottle up feelings that are hurting you deeply. Exposing it to trusted friends and relatives is an excellent healing method.

One of my close relatives called me on the phone weeping. He had failed one of his courses and felt very bad he had to rewrite it. Similarly, situations have caused many others to commit suicide. This happens mostly when there is no available shoulder to cry on. It is terrible when someone is facing challenges without any succoring empathy.

In the case of my relative, I shared his pain and encouraged him the best way I could. Although we were a great distance apart, I frequent calls and text messages to ensure he was fine and not attempting to hurt himself. It was difficult for him, but he got through it anyway. Today, he encourages people with his story. Indeed, what happens today becomes a history tomorrow.

Engage in Purposeful Activities

Tasks or behaviors with a well-defined aim or target are essentially purposeful. These are deliberate actions that provide a person's life purpose and fulfilment. These activities range from daily chores like washing the laundry or preparing meals to more important endeavors like volunteering or pursuing a passion or career. The important thing is that these pursuits are meaningful to the person seeking them and have a purpose.

One advantage of using meaningful activities to overcome depression is that they give a person's life structure and regularity. Finding the drive or energy to accomplish anything can be difficult for someone who is depressed. It is easier to get out of bed and begin the day positively if you have a list of meaningful things to partake in. This can give you a feeling of direction and purpose.

In addition, intentional actions might operate as a diversion from unfavourable emotions and ideas. People are less prone to dwell on their issues and concerns when concentrating on a task or objective. This can assist in ending the vicious cycle of pessimism that frequently accompanies depression.

Purposeful activity can also increase a person's sense of value and self-esteem. People feel pride and success when they complete tasks and reach their objectives. This can be especially helpful for those who are depressed because it can offset feelings of inferiority and worthlessness.

Another important advantage is the sense of social connection and belonging that purposeful activities foster. Depression can cause people to withdraw from society, which might make them feel disconnected and alone. However, purposeful activity makes it easier for people to interact with people who have similar interests. These activities undoubtedly promote a sense of community and lessen feelings of loneliness.

Being purpose-driven can assist people in finding new interests and passions, as sadness frequently causes people to lose interest in once-enjoyable activities. People could discover something that piques their attention and restore joy to their lives by attempting new things.

It is crucial to remember that participating in meaningful activities does not entail forcing oneself to perform tasks that are too difficult or overwhelming. It all comes down to balancing and selecting worthwhile and doable pursuits. Setting reasonable goals and avoiding putting undue strain on oneself is also critical. Finding pursuits that provide delight and a sense of purpose is the aim— not adding to the strain and stress.

Purposeful activity also offers social connection, organization, diversion, a sense of accomplishment, and the chance to explore new interests. It might not be a panacea for depression, but it can be a valuable tool for controlling symptoms and enhancing mental health in general. Therefore, if you or someone you know is experiencing depression, think about adding meaningful activities to your daily schedule. At the same time, you seek out professional assistance to create a customized rehabilitation plan.

Consider Medication

I used to know a particular lady who couldn't continue her tertiary education. She was depressed.

She stopped attending classes and failed to write assignments, tests, and exams. What worsened the matter was that she pretended to be okay and hid her feelings from anyone who could be helpful.

She didn't want to seek professional help or even take medication. Close friends and relatives had to force her to visit a medical practitioner. But they couldn't keep forcing her because she didn't embrace assistance. Eventually, she shut everyone out of her life. Sadly, her condition deteriorated.

In some instances, medication may be necessary to manage depression. Apart from just seeking professional aid, antidepressants prescribed by health practitioners can help alleviate symptoms. Adviseably, individuals suffering from depression should seek professional guidance before taking any medication.

Overcoming depression is a gradual process that requires dedication and perseverance. Seeking professional aid, practicing self-care, challenging negative thoughts, cultivating a support system, engaging in meaningful activities, practicing mindfulness, and considering medication when essential are crucial strategies. With the proper support and approaches, conquering depression is possible, paving the way for a fulfilling life. Always remember, there's hope for a brighter future and support available to navigate through these challenging times.

CHAPTER 6

Rediscovering Purpose

Finding your purpose again is one of the most life-changing experiences you can have when recovering from depression. People who are entangled in the darkness of despair frequently have a deep sensation of emptiness, as if the very core of who they are has been taken away. Reviving our sense of purpose, however, may light the road to healing and give our ideas, deeds, and interpersonal connections fresh vitality.

There is hope because you are still alive; it is not over yet. You can make sense out of life regardless of the terrible experiences you've had. The wonderful and ugly circumstances you've been through can become raw materials for producing a purposeful life.

Understanding Purpose

A wide definition of purpose is having a feeling of purposeful direction in life. It is the motivation behind our deeds and the lighthouse that leads us through life's challenges. This feeling of purpose can take many different forms, such as engagement in the community, family responsibilities, artistic pursuits, and professional goals. In the end, it is particular to each person and formed by their own experiences, values, and beliefs.

This feeling of direction might go lost when dealing with sadness. Something that was once inspiring and important might become insignificant, trapping people in a never-ending circle of pessimism. The good news is that purpose need not be a static idea; one may rediscover and renew it even in the most difficult times in life.

Why You Must Rediscover Purpose

Finding your purpose again may be a potent remedy for the hopelessness and loneliness that melancholy frequently brings on. Studies have indicated that participation in meaningful activities is associated with reduced levels of anxiety and depression, enhanced mental health outcomes, and heightened stress tolerance.

Steps to Rediscover Your Purpose

1. **Reflect on Your Values**: Think about what is most important to you to start. Which moral principles have guided your life, and which traits do you find admirable in others? Take note of them and search for any repeating themes or patterns. You might gain important insights from this thinking about potential areas of emphasis for your energy.

2. **Reconnect with Passions**: Recall the past pursuits you enjoyed. Resuming these hobbies—whether it was writing, painting,

gardening, or participating in sports—can inspire happiness and zeal. Reintroduce these hobbies into your daily life by starting small.

3. **Set Small Goals**: Start with attainable, reasonable objectives rather than taking on ambitious life ambitions. These might be as easy as reading a book chapter per week or as involved as giving a few hours a month. Reaching modest objectives may rekindle your enthusiasm and provide impetus for more ambitious ambitions.

4. **Seek Connection**: Interact with others who have similar beliefs or interests. In addition to offering support and motivation, social ties may provide people a feeling of community, which is essential for anybody overcoming depression. Go to support groups, meetings, or workshops to locate people who share your path.

5. **Practice Gratitude**: Taking stock of your life's blessings might help you change your perspective from one of hopelessness to one of opportunity. Think about keeping a thankfulness notebook in which you jot down any small acts of kindness you encounter on a daily or monthly basis. By doing this, you may change the way you think and become more aware of the worth that is all around you and inside you.

6. **Embrace Change**: Recognize that your goals could change in the future. Novel insights might arise from life events, human development, and evolving values. Be willing to try out new positions, interests, and pursuits. Accepting change may be freeing and open doors to unanticipated opportunities for happiness.

Finding your purpose again may seem like an impossible goal while you're depressed, but it's an essential first step on the road to recovery. You may put out the overpowering darkness by rekindling a flame of optimism by exploring your values, passions, and relationships. While purpose does not make grief go away, it may act as the catalyst for development, resiliency, and eventually healing.

Just as healing is progressive, remember that reclaiming your sense of purpose is a gradual process– one filled with self-discovery, vulnerability, and growth. Embrace the journey, trust in the process, and allow the rays of hope to guide you back to yourself.

CHAPTER 7

SUPPORT THE AILING

Our world is inundated with circumstances that inflict deep wounds in people's hearts. Both physical and social environments contribute to the kind and intensity of emotional pain individuals can suffer. As social beings, strengthening the weak and encouraging the broken-hearted are crucial to our peaceful coexistence.

Aiding the recovery of those experiencing depression through any helpful medium is vital. Doing this has two-way implications: first, the one who needs a cure gradually finds healing; second, the one who gives care strengthens their emotional resilience. You save a soul by encouraging people facing difficult times or considering calling it quits. Consequently, you are erecting a wall against emotional trauma.

After empowering others to smile, you will hardly feel sorrowful. As you radiate positive emotions toward others, your immunity against life's negative forces strengthens.

Noticeably, people who don't associate with others lose on both ends. They are weak emotionally and can hardly help anyone going through challenges.

Be Compassionate

Virtually everything we do begin with our mental construct. If you develop a positive mindset towards people, helping those in trauma becomes a natural flow. But those who create a social disconnect from society become critical and judgmental about other people.

Amazingly, when you decide to make a positive impact, the resources to actualize your resolve will gradually surface. Many people tie social relevance to financial buoyancy alone. But that's not true. Rich but unconcerned folks have low societal value.

You don't need money to encourage someone going through a tough time. All it requires is a heart of compassion and love. In fact, several rich people are tired of living. Money does not give them the happiness, sense of fulfillment, and meaning they desire. Such people do not need money to find healing.

Don't wait until you have all the wealth, resources, and riches you desire before you reach out compassionately to those going through difficult situations. With a compassionate heart, you can save a soul.

You may not have access to everyone in society, but you can brighten the corner where you are. You can give the world a smile. Your positive impact can begin within your circle of influence. Right where you are, someone possibly needs emotional support.

Compassion is a bridge that connects people. If everyone develops compassion and empathy, several social, financial, and emotional gaps will be filled. Instead of looking away from someone dying emotionally or criticizing them, you can be a source of strength and a beacon of hope.

Don't be judgmental

One of the easiest things to do is judge others and draw conclusions about them. However, assumption has been described as the lowest level of knowledge. We must never base our judgment of people's predicaments on our perceptions alone. Even if your perception is true, compassion can make you less judgmental.

Sometimes, we fail to help certain people because of our judgment. However, we may not always be correct. Some situations can hardly be understood or believed. I read of Joseph, who was wrongly accused of attempting rape. He was imprisoned for no just cause. This means that not everyone in prison is a criminal.

Some circumstances do not permit people to defend themselves. Only the report of others is taken to be true. In the case of Joseph, it was difficult for Potiphar to disbelieve his wife's allegation against the young boy. In reality, who should he believe: his wife or a slave?

Anyone in a situation where their explanations cannot be validated can tell the pain of being wrongly judged. Lousy judgment can aggravate people's pain or heighten their sorrows. When an individual finds that no one understands his situation, he feels isolated and lonely. This can worsen their emotional condition.

Not every accused is genuinely guilty, not all prisoners are criminals, and not everyone hanging on a cross is a thief. Therefore, we must be careful not to judge people wrongly because they face difficulties. You might need a total understanding of what led to their predicament.

Some challenging situations are transitional phases in people's lives. When such people overcome their challenges, they will remember those who stood by or scorned them.

Several people committed suicide because no one seemed to understand what they were going through. Some could not confide in anyone for fear of being misunderstood. You may be disappointed in someone for acting in a particular way, but learn not to abandon them in their trauma. You might be their final hope.

As a rule of thumb, don't conclude anything if you have no evidential backup. Learn not to be hasty in judging others. Cultivate the patience to listen to others without prejudice or misconception. You are healing the ailing souls by providing a shoulder others can lean on.

Reach Out

Today, almost everyone is engrossed in their activities. Looking out for other people's welfare is increasingly difficult. Daily, we all have more and more tasks and situations to deal with. However, we need other people just as they need us.

Occasionally, try to reach out to those around you, especially the ones who are going through difficult situations. A check-up call or visit can go a long way in alleviating their emotional pain. Checking up on people makes them feel loved and valued.

Reaching out to people around you to see how they are faring is a great act of love. It increases their confidence in you. When such people are experiencing emotional trauma, they will be more comfortable sharing their ordeals with you.

If you notice a change in the behavior of someone close to you, kindly contact them. They might be internally displaced. Don't assume they want to dissociate from you.

Some people experiencing depression may act strangely or ill-mannered. Please don't cut off from them because of that. If they had been well-behaved, something must have gone wrong with them. Create an opportunity for a harmless dialogue. You may be surprised at their response.

CONCLUSION

As we approach the end of Reigniting Hope: Your Exit from Depression, it is important to understand that this journey is about nourishing the source of hope that each of us possesses, not just about conquering an illness. Depression frequently has the sense of an unending storm, obscuring our best memories and sowing doubt in our brains. However, as we have seen, hope is a tenacious flame that may be kindled again, even in the direst circumstances.

We've x-rayed the complexities of depression and found methods and resources to turn hopelessness into possibilities. Every step taken toward recovery, from accepting self-compassion and making relationships to establishing routines and getting treatment from professionals, adds to the overall picture of recovery. This book is an invitation to go into the depths of your own creativity and resilience, not merely a compilation of methods.

I implore you to cling to the idea of a joyful, meaningful existence as you finish this book. Recognize that the road to recovery is a convoluted one with peaks and troughs rather than a straight one. It's acceptable to make mistakes and to ask for assistance when things get hard. Allow yourself to be receptive to the experiences, networks of support, and anecdotes that will help shed more light on your journey toward healing, just as you learned how to rekindle hope.

Recall that you are not alone yourself. Community, whether it comes from family, friends, or support groups, is a potent healing force. Let your voice be heard by sharing your victories and difficulties. Every interaction and dialogue has the power to uplift you and other people, spreading understanding and optimism.

Bring the insights you have gained, the affirmations, and the practical activities with you. Use them as instruments in your toolbox, prepared to be recalled at the first sign of uncertainty or gloom. You have a chance to cultivate self-love and kindness every day and take charge of your own mental health.

Accept the idea that there are countless opportunities ahead of you when you venture out into the world beyond these pages. Even on the cloudiest of days, your capacity to nurture hope will shine through the shadows of despair. Move forth with bravery, understanding that every day is a blank canvas filled with the vivid hues of your potential.

Let me conclude by reminding you that hope is a decision, an action, and a journey. Let's keep stoking the embers of potential, resiliency, and rejuvenation together. Remain brave, have faith in your own abilities, and never undervalue the influence of optimism. Even when the sunset is fading, a fresh beginning is always promising with every morning. Your narrative is not finished yet; the most captivating parts are still to come.